I0083589

Low Fodmap Diet

The Comprehensive Guide To Alleviating The Symptoms
Of IBS And Other Digestive Disorders With Numerous
Delicious And Healthy Gut-friendly Recipes

(The Methods For Treating IBS And Digestive Disorders)

Nathaniel Latham

TABLE OF CONTENT

Introduction

Irritable bowel syndrome accounts for roughly fifty percent of all digestive discomfort. Those affected daily experience symptoms including flatulence, diarrhea, constipation, bloating, and abdominal pain. In Europe, between 7 and 210 percent of the population is affected, with twice as many females as males. Because the disease is difficult to diagnose, it is frequently undiagnosed.

The bad news is that irritable bowel syndrome is incurable. The good news is that there is a way to significantly lessen the pain. The best part is that you have control and do not need to rely on medication.

Irritable bowel syndrome is caused by FODMAPs, or sugars with a short chain. With the low-FODMAP diet, the villains can be put in their place.

You are responsible for your own health. This book will assist you in identifying FODMAPs and eliminating them from your diet without sacrificing enjoyment.

Before beginning, you should consult your physician. Your symptoms may be indicative of a condition unrelated to irritable bowel syndrome. With a diagnosis or suspicion that your symptoms are due to a bowel irritation, you can begin treatment.

You will first gain a basic understanding of irritable bowel syndrome, its causes, and treatment options. This is followed by a 2 8 -day nutrition plan, and then the tasty part: 400 simple, delicious recipes that make it easier to change your diet. Best wishes on your journey towards irritable bowel syndrome relief!

Chapter 1: Does Irritable Bowel Syndrome Cause Joint Pain?

Did you know that if you have rheumatoid arthritis, you have an increased risk of developing gastrointestinal problems like irritable bowel syndrome (IBS)? A recent study found that those with rheumatoid arthritis had at least a 10 0% higher risk of developing a cardiovascular problem than those without the condition.

You may wonder how two seemingly unrelated conditions are connected. The reality, however, is that these two subjects are extremely interconnected.

Arthritis can significantly impact your daily life. Even after flushing the toilet, brushing your hair or urinating can be difficult. In the short term, arthritis medications treat the symptoms, but for long-term relief, addressing the cause of the condition is necessary. And that is why, if you have arthritis, you may be able to reduce inflammation and pain by enhancing your gut health.

What Is The Connection Between Rheumatoid Arthritis And Digestive Health?

There Are Several Reasons Why Those With Rheumatoid Arthritis Are More Likely To Experience Digestive Problems, Including Systemic Inflammation, Unbalanced Gut Bacteria, And An Increased Risk Of Developing Other Autoimmune Diseases Such As Celiac Disease And Crohn's Disease. As You May Be Aware, Approximately 210

Percent Of Those Diagnosed With An Autoimmune Disease Go On To Develop Others.

When The Gut Microbiome Is Out Of Whack And In A State Of Dysbiosis — In Which There Are More Opportunistic And Harmful Bacteria Than Beneficial Bacteria — It Can Trigger Inflammation In The Gut And Throughout The Body. Inflammation In The Gut May Cause Irritable Bowel Syndrome And Lead To Inflammation Of The Joints, A Symptom Of Rheumatoid Arthritis.

Studies Indicate That The Type Of Bacteria Residing In The Gut May Be Associated With The Incidence Of Rheumatoid Arthritis. Prevotella Copri Is A Type Of Bacteria That Stimulates The Release Of Specific Immune Cells That Cause Inflammation And An Inflammatory Pathway Associated With Rheumatoid Arthritis. Increased Abundance Of Prevotella Sorr In The

Intestines Is Also Associated With Irritable Bowel Syndrome Symptoms.

Chapter 2: Should You Follow A Low-Fodmap Diet?

It is essential to understand that IBS and other functional bowel disorders are not caused by consuming FODMAPs; therefore, eliminating FODMAPs from the diet will not cure a disease or disorder. A low FODMAP diet aims to reduce digestive symptoms by eliminating high FODMAP foods and replacing them with low FODMAP alternatives. This diet may not be suitable for everyone. It is intended to be a short-term diet and is typically adhered to for two weeks or less. It should not be used as a long-term diet solution. Consult your healthcare provider prior to beginning a low FODMAP diet in order to eliminate other causes of your symptoms. Low FODMAP diets have proven to be most beneficial for those with:

• An offsal dagno of Irrtable Bowel Sundrome (IBS), Inflammatoru Bowel Deae (IBD), or other funstonal bowel dorder with symptoms of excessive gas, bloat, abdominal pain, diarrhea/constipation, etc.

• Tried and failed standard therapy (high-carbohydrate diet, increased fluid intake, increased physical activity, etc.).

• A terrible calamity has been ruled out as improbable. The removal of wheat from the diet will affect the accuracy of future seliometric testing.

Regular Or Irregular Consumption Of High Fodmap Food The desire and capacity to modify their diet.

FODMAP Elimination diet:

A FODMAP elimination sonata with three stanzas:

• Elimination protocol: all FODMAPs are eliminated from the diet for two to six weeks.

• Challenge phase: the body is challenged by reintroducing FODMAPs into the diet in a systematic manner. Symptoms are preserved and FODMAP-related problems are identified.

• Final phase: problem FODMAPs are assimilated into the diet and tolerated.

10

Allow the Helr of a Registered Dodecanese:

If it is determined that a low FODMAP diet would be beneficial for you, consulting with a Registered Dietitian (RD) who specializes in gastroenterological nutrition will increase your likelihood of success. The RD will help identify major FODMAP sulrrt in your diet and develop an individualized diet plan based on your eating habits and food preferences in order to improve your symptoms and quality of life. In an attempt to alleviate symptoms, individuals are often overly restrictive with their diet. This resulted in nutritional deficiency. The purpose of the FODMAP diet is to manage symptoms while allowing for the most varied and nutritious diet possible.

Chapter 3 : It Is Possible To Consume A Tasty Low-Fodmap Diet

Garlic and onions contain a high amount of FODMAPs. Consequently, the misconception that a low-FODMAP diet is flavorless has grown.

While many recipes call for fresh onion and garlic, there are numerous herbs, spices, and flavorings that are low in FODMAPs that can be substituted.

Additionally, simple using garlic-infused oil that is low in FODMAPs and filtered will still impart garlic flavor. The garlic absorbs the flavor of the oil, but not the FODMAPs, since garlic does not contain fat-soluble FODMAPs.

Chapter 4: The Axis Of The Gut And Brain And Gut Sensitivity

In the intestinal walls of the gastrointestinal (GI) tract are neural circuits, which are nerves. The Enteric Nervous System (ENS) is a large, complex network of nerves that controls the gut's response to food by regulating digestion, intestinal motility (how quickly food moves through the intestines), nutrient absorption, and waste elimination.

Gut Brain Dysfunction occurs when the Gut Brain Axis is out of balance due to factors such as chronic daily life stressors, early life trauma, anxiety (both general and anticipated IBS symptom anxiety), and depression.

Gut Brain Dysfunction can lead to communication difficulties between the gut and brain, which can result in a highly sensitive gut wall. Visceral Hypersensitivity is the condition in which the Enteric Nervous System sends stronger pain signals to the brain in response to normal digestion characteristics such as food movement through the GI tract, bloating, and gas. These normally unnoticed aspects of digestion are experienced as painful, uncomfortable symptoms. It is believed that approximately 60% of IBS patients have a hypersensitive gut wall.

Spend Some Time Familiarizing Yourself With The Diet

Spend some time familiarizing yourself with the low-FODMAP diet before beginning. Consult a dietitian or doctor for advice, and then conduct online research. Determine which foods you can consume and which you should avoid. Consider recipes that are low in FODMAPs.

Without adequate preparation, beginning a low FODMAP diet can result in errors and be extremely frustrating. The optimal strategy is to prepare yourself.

2. SEEK OUT A FODMAP-CERTIFIED NUTRITION PROFESSIONAL

The FODMAP diet is difficult to adhere to. In the beginning, it is easy to make mistakes. It is essential to get all the nutrients you need and to avoid a strict low-FODMAP diet for an extended period of time.

To properly adhere to the diet, assistance from a dietitian who has completed a FODMAP certification program is essential.

AVOID FODMAPS STACKING The practice of eating multiple items from the same FODMAP group at once is known as FODMAP stacking. Although they may be low in FODMAPs when consumed individually, consuming them all at once could cause you to exceed your FODMAP limit. This may cause symptoms.

8 . AVOID SIMPLE USING LARGE SERVINGS

The FODMAP diet focuses solely on portion sizes. There are numerous limited-quantity foods that are low in FODMAPs. For example, 60 grams of zucchini contain very few or no FODMAPs. However, a 2 00-gram serving of zucchini is rich in fructans. This may result in symptoms.

Consequently, it is essential to review and adhere to the low FODMAP serving sizes for each product.

Additionally, eating excessively and consuming large portions of food may cause IBS symptoms. Therefore, it is essential to control your portion sizes.

Chapter 6: What To Enter Into Your Food Diary

For the duration of the final phase of your eating regimen, monitor your indicators. Observe characteristics such as internal tendencies, torment, and bulging. Here is an example of what can be recorded. You may also rate the response on a scale from 2 to 2 0 based on the severity of symptoms after eating (2 being fine, 2 0 being extreme). Simple using the accompanying templates, maintain a daily journal that will allow you to track your reaction to the low FODMAP diet.

Once your symptoms are under control and you are beginning the reintroduction phase, keep track of the foods and quantities you reintroduce.

Then, record any manifestations you experience at that time. In light of your reaction and resistance to the test foods, you should be able to determine the source of your symptoms. For instance, if you experience an outbreak of pain, excessive wind, or a change in your internal tendencies, you will be able to determine which food caused it.

What Are Fodmaps?

"FODMAP" is an acronym for "fermentable oligo-, disaccharides, and polyols."

These nondigestible short-shank sardines are osmotically active, which means they draw water into the digestive tract. In addition, because they are indigestible, your gut bacteria ferment them, resulting in an increase in gas and short-chain fatty acid production. Therefore, FODMAPs are notorious for casimple using digestive symptoms such as bloating, gas, diarrhea, or a combination of the two. Approximately sixty percent of IBS patients have reported that fasting worsens or worsens their symptoms. FODMAPs are present in varying amounts in a variety of foods. Some foods contain only one variety, while others contain several. Oligosaccharides include wheat, rye, nuts, legumes, artichokes, and onions. Dassharde: lastoe-sontanng rrodust such as milk, yogurt, soft cheese, ice cream, buttermilk, sour milk, and whipped cream * Monoassharde: foods containing fructose, such as apples, pears, watermelons, and mango, as well as sweeteners such as honey, agave nectar, and high fructose corn syrup. Polyols: mannitol and sorbitol in asparagus, broccoli, cauliflower, shiijust take mushrooms, and snow peas, as well as xylitol and isomalt in low-calorie sweeteners like sugar-free gum and mints.

Chapter 7: Why People Become Vegans

First, let's establish a few definitions so that there are no ambiguities. In general, '-m' refers to a belief item, while '-aran' refers to the role that follows it. However, this is not always the case, as being a "humanitarian" does not imply that you enjoy eating human flesh with your salad. Vegetaran do not eat any meat, though some eat fresh egg fresh fresh egg and daru rrodust, whereas vegan abstain from all anmal or bu-rrodust and refuse to consume even honey or butter.

The top three reasons why people choose to be vegan are as follows:

– Animal rights Vegans believe animals have the right to live without human interference.

– The atmosphere Animal feed production uses a great deal of land, fertilizer, and water that could be used to feed people. It is believed that lvetosk rroduston accelerates torol oxidation, thereby decreasing t rrodustvtu for the production of sulfur. Animal waste also causes sedimentation in groundwater and rivers.

– Personal health Going vegan increases one's energy, aids in weight loss, and helps maintain a healthy weight and youthful appearance.

The ethical reasons are the most intriguing, especially in cases where individuals are adamantly opposed to eating animal products but do not adhere to a plant-based diet. The farming of some exotic foods can cause significant ethical problems, such as with the soy farms that are deforesting the Amazon or the pesticides used on fresh bananas by the Dole Corporation, resulting in infertility among the workers. If you are not cautious, you should be consuming wild animals while killing humans. Therefore, if you truly want to be an ethical vegan, you must reearch all of your food, including the rlant.

On the other side of the vegan dilemma are meat eaters who are unaware that veganism has been proven to be extremely healthy. Too often in Afrisan sosieties todau, meat eaters mosk vegetarians and vegans. The most common anti-vegan/vegetarian argument made by omnivores (those who eat both meat and vegetables) is that humans cannot obtain enough protein from vegetables alone. This is a moth: Vegetables, in all their glory, provide all the vital nutrients a human needs to survive, when consumed in the proper manner.

If veganism resulted in malnutrition, many non-meat-eating cultures and societies would perish. Also, half of Holluwood would be dead (here, half of Holluwood would be vegetarian). For example, the film's male lead, Lam Hemsworth, is a well-known actor. The Hunger Games, without mentioning the first word of the film's title. Hr-hor rroduser Ruell Smmon and ror nger Arana Grande also live a parallel existence. Rarrer Waska Floska Flame (see him making vegan blueberru muffins here) went vegan to avoid besoming fat. Athletes such as Carl Lewy would not have won an Olympic gold medal (see his video on winning an Olympic gold medal as a vegan).

Pre-solunar Africans subsisted predominately on a rlant-based diet. Alan Levne/Flskr/CC photo

Even the Bible is in favor of veganism. This is where the annual 'Danel Fat' song gathering, practiced by many Christians, originates:

"However, Daniel resolved that he would not deplete himself with food and drink... Then Daniel asked ... "Give you vegetables to eat and water to drink"... At the conclusion of ten days, it was observed that you were healthier and fatter than all the young men who had been eating the roast rooster." – Daniel 2 :8, 2 2 –2 2, 2 10

Numerous sentfs evdense the benefits of a rredomnantly plant-based diet, ranging from the prevention of scurvy to a more enjoyable eating experience.

Chapter 8: Overview Of Ibs And The Low-Fodmap Diet

An IBS-Overview

Irritable bowel syndrome (IBS) is a common digestive disorder affecting approximately 2 10 % of the population. Various ages of men and women are affected. Symptoms include excessive flatulence, abdominal distension, pain or discomfort, and altered bowel habits (diarrhea, constipation, or a combination of both). These symptoms vary in intensity from day to day and week to week. Due to the fact that IBS is diagnosed based on the pattern of symptoms, it is essential to rule out other disorders with similar symptoms, such as celiac disease and inflammatory bowel disease (IBD), which may be mistaken for IBS. Before beginning a low-FODMAP or gluten-free diet, everyone with IBS symptoms should be evaluated for these conditions, so if you haven't already, consult your physician about getting tested. However, keep in mind that IBS can coexist with other digestive diseases.

FODMAPS PRODUCE IBS FODMAPs share the following characteristics:

The absorption rate in the small intestine is low. This suggests that many of these molecules bypass the small intestine and travel directly to the colon without being absorbed. This is due to their inability to be metabolized and delayed absorption. Our capacity to digest and absorb various FODMAPs differs among individuals: Some people do not produce enough lactase (the enzyme required to break down lactose), and the capacity to absorb polyols (which are the wrong shape to pass easily through the small intestinal lining) also varies from person to person. No one can digest fructans and galactooligosaccharides (GOS), so they are poorly absorbed by everyone.

They are tiny molecules that are consumed in large quantities. When molecules are poorly absorbed, the body attempts to "dilute" them by pumping water into the gastrointestinal system. The presence of excess fluid in the digestive system can cause diarrhea and interfere with the gut's muscular activity.

They are "fast food" for the naturally occurring bacteria in the large intestine. There are billions of bacteria in the large intestine (and the bottom section of the small intestine). If chemicals are not absorbed in the small intestine, they reach the large intestine. These food molecules are considered rapid food by the local bacteria, and they are rapidly broken down to produce hydrogen, carbon dioxide, and methane. The chain length determines the rate at which molecules ferment: Unlike fiber, which consists of molecules with significantly longer chain lengths known as polysaccharides, oligosaccharides, and simple sugars ferment relatively rapidly. In the majority of meals, numerous FODMAPs are present. Until they reach the lower small intestine and colon, their effects are cumulative, as they all produce distension in the same manner. This indicates that the degree of intestinal distension is determined by the total amount of FODMAPs consumed, as opposed to the amount of each individual FODMAP. Suppose a person with difficulty digesting lactose and absorbing fructose consumes a meal containing lactose. In this case, fructans, polyols, GOS, and fructose will have an effect on the intestine that is $2 + 2 + 2 + 2 + 2 = 10$ times greater than if they consumed the same amount of a single FODMAP. Consequently, we must consider all FODMAPs when altering our diet.

FODMAPs are a group of naturally occurring sugars that are not absorbed in the small intestine; instead, they travel to the large intestine, where bacteria are present (which is normal and healthy). These bacteria utilize FODMAPs (unabsorbed sugars) as a food source. When bacteria consume FODMAPs, they ferment them, which can result in excessive flatulence, gassiness, bloating, abdominal distension, and abdominal pain. In susceptible individuals, FODMAPs can also alter the rate at which the bowels move, leading to constipation, diarrhea, or a combination of both. It is evident that FODMAPs trigger IBS symptoms.

All of the recipes in this book contain ingredients that are low in FODMAPs, excluding those that are high in FODMAPs (see table on facing page).

WHEN SHOULD AN INDIVIDUAL CONSIDER THE LOW FODMAP DIET?

The Low FODMAP diet is not suitable for everyone. It is intended to aid those with stomach-related infections in their recovery. Four organs comprise the stomach-related framework: the GI (gastrointestinal tract), liver, gallbladder, and pancreas. Any issue with these areas indicates an issue with the stomach. This is concerning not only because it renders life hopeless, but also because it places your immune system in jeopardy. 80 percent of your immune system is located in the stomach. Stomach illnesses can be either temporary or persistent. The following are three stomach-related conditions that the Low FODMAP diet can effectively treat:

Crohn's illness

Constant in nature, Crohn's disease is characterized by gastrointestinal inflammation. It typically attacks the small intestine and an internal organ, but any portion of the body (from the mouth to the buttocks) can be affected. Usually, it begins with mild symptoms and progressively worsens over time, but it can go into remission for years or even decades.

Symptoms include weight loss, stomach pain and constriction, diarrhea, sickness, fatigue, joint pain, and nausea, among others. According to research, the manifestations of eczema vary depending on the site of irritation, and stress can exacerbate the symptoms. Certain food sources can also irritate the digestive system and exacerbate symptoms.

Over 10 00,000 Americans suffer from Crohn's disease. If you are between 20 and 29 years old, smoke, or have a family member with Crohn's disease, you will develop the disease. Experts are unsure of the precise cause of Crohn's disease, but they have a few hypotheses. It may be caused by an immune system response, which occurs when your immune system attacks your digestive system and solid cells, misjust taking them for the enemy.

Low FODMAP Diet Menu

We understand that planning low FODMAP meals can be intimidating, especially if you were recently diagnosed with irritable bowel syndrome (IBS) and are new to the FODMAP diet. Here are some of our kitchen organization tips and a sample low FODMAP meal plan to help you prepare in advance.

Tips for FODMAP-friendly meal planning

Do not believe that you must completely alter your diet. Instead, consider the meals that you typically enjoy (such as spaghetti bolognaise or Thai green curry) and how they could be modified by substituting IBS-triggering foods with low FODMAP alternatives. Gluten-free alternatives and olive oils infused with garlic are excellent replacements for those who fear giving up wheat and garlic-based products.

During step 2 of the FODMAP diet, educate yourself on label reading and how to identify FODMAPs in packaged foods so that you can shop with confidence.

Spend some time on the weekend writing down your weekly meal plans (either on paper, in your phone's notes, or even on a whiteboard), and then create your FODMAP shopping list.

Preparing some healthy low FODMAP meals in advance (Sundays are typically a good day for this) is also an excellent way to stay organized and avoid the stress of easily cooking or coming up with meal ideas during the week. So many delectable meals can be easily frozen and are a time-saver in the future.

Check out the Monash FODMAP recipe page if you need low FODMAP recipe inspiration. This book has more recipes than our app (due to the app's limited storage capacity) and is full of family-friendly options.

Chapter 9: Changing The Diet And Way Of Life Is The Primary Treatment For Ibs.

Consuming small servings 10 -6 times daily. Food should be served neither too hot nor too cold.

Just take brief breaks in between meals.

Consume nothing before bedtime.

Establish a regular eating schedule (breakfast, lunch, and dinner, with snacks as needed) and avoid skipping meals or just taking long breaks between meals.

Avoid consuming large quantities of food and thoroughly chew your food.

Avoid consuming alcoholic beverages and tobacco products.

• Oats (soluble dietary fiber) in cereals and cereals, as well as flax seeds, can reduce bloating (up to one tablespoon per day).

If you have diarrhea or flatulence, limit your injust take of fresh fruits to no more than three servings per day (80 g each).

No sweeteners should be utilized.

If you suffer from abdominal bloating, you should reduce your consumption of cabbage, whole milk, and flour products.

For constipation, increase the amount of fiber consumed (fiber absorbs water, which normalizes the stool and reduces pain spasms) and monitor the amount of fluid consumed.

Many intestinal complaints disappear when a person begins to drink more water, especially if they have IBS with constipation. Even if you do not go outside or feel thirsty, the World Health Organization recommends that you drink at least six glasses of water per day (2 .10 liters). If you do not prefer cold water, you may consume warm water. Tea can be used in place of water.

Food ought to be boiled, steamed, or braised.

Participate in physical activity

● When possible, avoid stressful situations.

Fundamentals of Nutrition

Dietary recommendations for irritable bowel syndrome depend on the severity of symptoms and the underlying disease. The syndrome can result in pain, constipation, diarrhea, or flatulence, but the underlying principles are universal. A specialist will recommend an approximate diet and list of permitted foods.

The fundamental guidelines of the IBS diet are as follows:

Consistent but moderate food consumption. You must eat promptly because you cannot be late for your next appointment. If someone is at work, you are required to easily bring homemade food.

Meals should be eaten frequently - 8 -6 times per day in small portions. You should eat every 6 hours - this is the best option because you will not experience hunger, stomach fullness, or overeating.

Following a meal, you should wait three hours. To prevent indigestion and a worsening of painful symptoms, you should not fall asleep instantly. The food is light, with a focus on proteins.

Add liquid soups, cereals, and dairy products to the menu. Avoid fast food, spicy foods, fried foods, and fatty foods.

● You can keep a food journal and record all the ingredients you consume to determine the cause of the syndrome and the food that exacerbated it.

The patient must consume at least 2 liters of liquid per day, preferably purified water, gas-free mineral water, or dried fruit compotes. Nutritional guidelines must be followed. It is essential to maintain composure throughout therapy in order to resume the hourly diet.

Dietary nutrition is intended to alleviate uncomfortable symptoms. Dietary staples should consist of foods rich in dietary fiber.
Highlighted Products
Low-fat meals and foods high in protein, fiber, and carbohydrates are permitted for those with irritable bowel syndrome.

Broths made from low-fat vegetables, meat, and fish, porridge made from wheat, buckwheat, and barley just cooked just just cooked in water, dietary meat (beef, rabbit, nutria) in steam, boiled, and baked forms, crackers made from white wheat bread, vegetables (cauliflower, carrots), carefully thermally processed, baked apples, berry kissels, weak tea, rosehip broth effectively act on the body, low-fat dairy products (kefir, cottage cheese, homemade yogurt).

The list of acceptable products can be slightly narrowed or broadened based on the presence of symptoms and the unique characteristics of the organism.

Prohibited Merchandise
During illness, products that irritate the intestines, cause gas formation and fermentation, and stimulate peristalsis should be avoided.

Avoid the following fermentable foods: marinades, smoked meats, sausages, fresh fruits and vegetables, legumes, mushrooms, grapes, cabbage, and berries.

Condensed milk, candy, chocolate, strongly brewed tea, coffee, alcohol, soda, crackers, chips, fast foods, fatty meats (pork, lamb), semi-finished products, pastries, drinks containing gas, refined sugar.

This list should be taken seriously, and it can be expanded in cases of intolerance. If the recommendations are not adhered to, the syndrome will worsen and the pathological symptoms will become more complex.

It is important to note that therapeutic nutrition will vary depending on the manifestation of symptoms in adults.

What is IBS

A disorder of the digestive tract typically characterized by stomach pain, bloating, and alterations in gut tendencies. This may include diarrhea, obstruction, or both, with one occurring after the other. Additionally known as irritable colon, sensitive colon, bodily fluid colitis, and spastic colon.

IBS is a common condition affecting the gastrointestinal system. It is a common but awkward digestive issue. Irritable Bowel Syndrome (IBS) is surprisingly common. According to the overall data, the prevalence of IBS ranges between 2 0 and 26 percent. Many individuals with IBS are undiagnosed or unaware of their condition.

The cause(s) of IBS are currently unknown. Regardless, there are risk factors that can predispose an individual to IBS. In the following pages, we will examine each of these in detail.

Symptoms

Irritable bowel syndrome (IBS) is a common disorder affecting the stomach and digestive organs, also known as the gastrointestinal tract. Side effects include constriction, stomach pain, swelling, gas, and diarrhea or constipation, or both. IBS is a chronic condition that requires long-term management. IBS does not harm the digestive system or increase the risk of colon cancer. Frequently, side effects can be managed through dietary and lifestyle changes.

However, triggers vary from person to person, making it difficult to identify specific food sources or stressors that all affected individuals should avoid. There may be times when your side effects are more tolerable and times when they are more distressing (eruptions). They may be triggered by food or drink.

IBS can also result in:

farting (flatulence) (flatulence)

passing mucus from your genitalia fatigue and lack of energy feeling ill (nausea)

backache \sproblems urination, such as frequent urination, sudden urges to urinate, and the sensation that you cannot completely empty your bladder; inability to control when you defecate (bowel incontinence).

IBS pain is visceral discomfort. This indicates that it originates from an organ. In this case, the colon and intestines.

While the majority of IBS cases are mild to moderate, approximately 20% of cases are considered severe. IBS can last for several weeks or even months, whereas a typical stomachache only lasts a couple of days.

Irritable bowel syndrome can affect anyone, but it is twice as prevalent in women as in men. IBS is also more likely to affect individuals with a family history of the disorder. Symptoms typically manifest before the age of 6 10 . Rarely do people over 10 0 develop IBS for the first time.

Chapter 11: Fodmap Diet Several Stages Of The Diet

In the initial phase, you should adhere to a strict low-FODMAP diet. This phase should last between four and one and a half months. As a result of the drastic reduction in FODMAPs, you should observe an improvement in your symptoms. As long as this type of diet fails to alleviate your side effects, you cannot proceed to stage 2 of this eating plan. If necessary, you can extend the duration of the initial phase to approximately two months. If there is still no improvement after this time period, you should discontinue the diet. The source of your complaints may not be combated with this type of dietary modification.

Throughout the second phase of the diet, FODMAP-rich foods are gradually reintroduced. By gradually expanding your diet, you can more effectively determine which food sources are casimple using you symptoms and which food varieties your body can tolerate. Unfortunately, there is no conclusive answer as to which food sources your body can tolerate. If you experience side effects after consuming a particular food, you should avoid it in the future. You can also try eating this food again in a different combination in the future. It might not produce any effects. Then you will know how to enjoy this food in the future without experiencing any discomfort. The best course of action is to record the relative number of food sources you have tried and whether or not they triggered symptoms. The FODMAP-reduced menu will eventually incorporate all food varieties that do not cause symptoms.

In the third step, you create a single menu comprising the stage 2 list. If you adhere to this arrangement, you will be able to continue your normal daily activities with minimal side effects.

Chapter 12 : Low Fodmap Diet Guide For Ibs

Irritable bowel syndrome (IBS) is treated with a diet low in FODMAPs. This is one of the most common and commonly suggested treatments. If you have recently been diagnosed with irritable bowel syndrome (IBS) or are still awaiting confirmation of your diagnosis, it is likely that you have been advised to try the FODMAP diet.

Nevertheless, it is entirely possible that you have no idea what it means.

FODMAPs are fermentable oligosaccharides, disaccharides, monosaccharides, and polyols. These short-chain carbohydrates are difficult to digest, so the gut absorbs only a portion of them.

As a result of this characteristic, they are frequently considered to be potential causes of IBS symptoms. A diet low in FODMAP promotes the consumption of foods with a lower concentration of these carbohydrates.

Changing to a diet low in FODMAPs may be the most effective way to gain control over your irritable bowel syndrome symptoms, despite its difficulty. Before beginning, you must have a thorough understanding of what FODMAPs are, what they cause, and which foods contain them.

When you first begin to just take control of your IBS and manage it properly, you will frequently hear the term "FODMAP." Additionally, it may be difficult to comprehend.

To begin, let's examine the acronym's breakdown. The acronym FODMAP refers to fermentable oligosaccharides, disaccharides, monosaccharides, and polyols.

These are short-chain carbohydrates, and they are typically absorbed by the large intestine, where colonic bacteria ferment them into acetic acid.

Throughout the duration of the fermentation process, they just take in water and produce a significant amount of gas. These gases cause the gut to swell, resulting in a painful and distressing experience.

FODMAPs, both naturally occurring and added, may be problematic for individuals with digestive issues. Here is a list of foods that typically contain various FODMAPs:

Examples of foods that contain oligosaccharides are wheat, rye, garlic, onions, artichokes, and legumes.

Fruits and dairy products like milk and yogurt contain disaccharides.

Fruits, honey, and the nectar of the agave plant are all examples of monosaccharides.

Natural and artificial sweeteners, as well as fruits and vegetables, contain polyols.

Clearly, FODMAPs are present in a wide variety of foods. Therefore, adhering to a diet low in FODMAPs may be difficult. It is more important to determine which FODMAPs are casimple using your symptoms than to completely eliminate them from your diet.

Beginning a FODMAP-Restricted Diet

Understanding what FODMAPs are and what they do can make starting a new diet feel overwhelming. Because FODMAPs are found in so many food groups, it may seem impossible to completely eliminate them from one's diet.

Understanding that following a low-FODMAP diet is only a temporary consideration should be your first step. This diet has so few options that it is impossible to adhere to for an extended period.

The low-FODMAP diet consists of three distinct phases:

Phase 2 : The Elimination Procedure

In the initial phase of the diet, you will be required to eliminate all FODMAP-rich foods.

Depending on how quickly your symptoms begin to improve, this stage can last between three and eight weeks. If you continue to experience difficulties after eight weeks, you should consult a healthcare professional.

Before beginning the process of eliminating foods from your diet, always consult a nutritionist or medical professional to ensure that the diet is appropriate for your needs.

Reintroduction to the Population in Phase 2

After completing the elimination phase of IBS treatment and observing an improvement in symptoms, it is time to begin reintroducing foods into your diet.

The recommended course of action is to add one new meal to the diet every three to seven days while keeping a close eye on the symptoms. It is advised that you do this under the supervision of a dietitian.

The objective of the reintroduction phase of the elimination diet is to determine which foods you can tolerate and in what amounts. If symptoms appear, restart the elimination diet with the offending food, and when you feel better, attempt to reintroduce another food.

Stage 6 – Personalization

At the third stage, you will still need to limit your consumption of FODMAPs, but you will have a better understanding of which specific types trigger an adverse reaction. This stage is also known as the maintenance phase in some circles.

The diet will be very similar to normal, with the exception that high-FODMAP foods, which caused symptoms during the reintroduction period, will be excluded. It is possible that the diet will require further modification in the future.

Chapter 13: Different Phases Of The Fodmap Diet

In order to effectively manage symptoms, the Low FODMAP Diet entails a temporary reduction in FODMAP consumption.

In addition, the elimination is temporary.

The low FODMAP diet has three phases, not just elimination.

The low FODMAP elimination phase is the initial phase and involves reducing your overall FODMAP consumption.

Equal in significance are the remaining stages. During the first two to six weeks of the first phase, you consume only low FODMAP foods to help you control your symptoms and observe how you react.

In two to six weeks, the majority of patients will experience symptom relief;

however, some patients may require a little longer. Some dietitians may recommend that you extend the first phase of the low FODMAP diet to see if you can better manage your symptoms.

The second phase, reintroduction, consists primarily of gradually reintroducing FODMAP categories.

In order to determine how much FODMAPs you can tolerate in each category, we can use this information to determine how much we can gradually increase your consumption.

Depending on the frequency of your symptoms during reintroduction, the reintroduction phase can last anywhere from six to twelve weeks, and sometimes even longer.

The Low FODMAP Diet's third and final phase is liberalization.

In this section, we include foods that you have tolerated well in the quantities that you have tolerated. In addition, we occasionally include FODMAPs that you may not have tolerated well in small quantities or when your gut is healthy.

The ultimate goal is to have the most liberalized diet possible, so that you don't focus on the restrictive aspects of the diet and are less concerned about what you eat.

The objective is to ensure that we are as tolerant and food-loving as possible.

It is essential to comprehend that the Low FODMAP Diet is not all or nothing.

FODMAPs need not be completely eliminated from your diet for the rest of your life.

It boils down to this three-phase strategy. Moreover, it is acceptable to consume FODMAPs during the elimination or initial phase.

The consumption of these will not harm your stomach.

They will only possibly exhibit symptoms.

Simply observe how your body responds before returning to the low FODMAP diet as soon as possible. To maximize one's enjoyment of food and life, the ultimate objective is to maintain a varied diet.

FODMAP Subclasses

Lactose is the first classification.

Some individuals who have difficulty digesting lactose may experience bloating, diarrhea, or constipation when consuming dairy products.

Lactose is consumed through milk, yogurt, and cheese.

Dairy products are permitted on the Low FODMAP Diet.

Instead, it consists of a low lactose diet that allows dairy consumption.

Simply put, it must have a low lactose content.

This can therefore include lactose-free milk, lactose-free yogurt, and even hard cheeses, which contain little lactose by nature.

Thus, there is still a great deal of variety.

If you consume dairy, it is more important to make healthy choices within the dairy category than to give it up entirely.

The second category contains fructose.

Fruit sugar, also known as fructose, is a type of sugar found in fruits.

We all have a limited capacity for fructose absorption, so fructose in extremely high concentrations is difficult for everyone to absorb.

However, some individuals have difficulty absorbing even trace amounts of fructose.

It may draw water into the bowels, resulting in bloating, diarrhea, and the appearance of being stretched out.

Numerous fruits and vegetables contain fructose, including watermelon, apples, cherries, and pears, as well as asparagus, sugar snap peas, and broccoli stocks.

In addition to high fructose corn syrup and sweeteners such as honey and agave, it is also present in our confections.

Therefore, if you see these ingredients on the label, they are likely high in fructose and may cause gastrointestinal distress.

The third category consists of sugar alcohols.

The main sources of the sugars mannitol and sorbitol are our fruits and vegetables.

Thus, our fruits and vegetables with pits, including winter squash, artichokes, plums, nectarines, pit peaches, pit cherries, and pit avocados.

Additionally, it is used as a sugar substitute in numerous low-calorie, diabetic, and keto treats. Because it is poorly absorbed, it tastes sweet but contains no calories.

Check the labels of such foods, as they may cause diarrhea by drawing water into the intestines.

The fructans and GOS or LACTO oligosaccharides, which ferment rapidly in the intestine and cause a great deal of gas and bloating, were among the final categories to be merged.

They can also alter bowel habits.

Some fruits and vegetables contain them, especially onions and garlic.

These are relatively difficult to eliminate or reduce.

I would like you to be aware that foods such as fresh onion and garlic ferment in the gut and cause gastrointestinal distress.

In addition to other plant-based foods such as soy, it is also present in our wheat products, such as wheat, barley, and rye.

Soy milk, silken tofu, and various nuts and seeds, including cashews, pistachios, and almonds, are among the milk substitutes available.

How do we then determine which foods contain what amounts of FODMAPs?

I believe there is an outstanding app for that.

Extensive research has been conducted on the Low FODMAP Diet, and Monash University, which has paved the way for this diet, has developed an excellent app.

And YES, the ten dollars are worth every penny.

Additionally, virtually every type of food has been evaluated to determine its FODMAP content.

They use a traffic light system, so during the elimination phase, you can either adhere strictly to green foods or, as I frequently do, allow them to consume one yellow food per meal. And this has served me and many others well.

In addition, this is less restrictive and offers slightly more variety.

If this doesn't work for some reason, you can always just take a stricter approach.

Consequently, during the elimination phase, we should generally restrict ourselves to green foods.

Simply determine which portion sizes we can accommodate.

In this case, reintroduction reallly becomes relevant.

In conclusion, the Low FODMAP Diet can significantly reduce IBS symptoms such as gas, bloating, abdominal pain, and bowel habit changes, especially diarrhea.

According to the research, 10 0% to 710 % of patients benefit.

The Low FODMAP Diet is effective for a subset of these patients, but not all will experience symptom relief.

In addition, it is essential to be aware that, due to the fact that many individuals end up on a very restrictive diet, it can be difficult to implement correctly and safely.

Chapter 14: Vegans can commence the Low FODMAP Diet.

Low FODMAP is the scientific name given to the diet used to manage IBS symptoms, if you haven't heard of it before.

I have been a vegan for approximately ten years. But about four to six months ago, I went vegan and felt awful about my diet. I was dissatisfied with the diet because it did not match what I saw on the internet.

Therefore, I decided to begin the low fodmap diet. Later, I discovered that the low fodmap diet combined with the vegan diet was significantly superior to the vegan diet alone.

The low fodmap diet consists primarily of garlic, onions, and avocados.

There is very little information online about the low fodmap diet, particularly for those who wish to use it to treat IBS.

This is the reason I wrote this book: to provide you with ideas and recipes for managing IBS and gut problems.

I'm going to reveal a multitude of useful tips for this diet.

This book will also discuss the cultivation of a healthy microbiome, which consists of all the beneficial bacteria and viruses that reside in the body and work hard to support it.

One of the primary causes of your IBS is that the bacterial community in your stomach is out of balance.

Numerous significant studies have been conducted regarding the low fodmap diet. To completely heal IBS, you should begin incorporating some of these practices and lifestyles into your diet.

Note that the low fodmap diet only aids in the management of IBS. It is not a treatment. You will return to your normal diet in the long run. You are only on the low fodmap diet to assist in restoring balance to your bacterial community.

Chapter 15: Plant-Based Diet Low In Fodmaps

Plant-derived det

What do oranges, almonds, bay leaves, and cloves have in common with cinnamon? All of you are plants. This book will explain what a plant-based diet is, how to eat a plant-based low FODMAP diet, and how to incorporate more plants into your diet, whether or not you are following a low FODMAP diet.

A plant-based diet is one in which you consume primarily plants. It means that the majority of the foods you consume are plant-based, with the occasional addition of meat or dairy. It does not imply that you must be vegetarian or vegan, despite the fact that these are also rlant-based diets. The emphasis is on consuming and appreciating an abundance of vegetables, nuts, seeds, legumes, whole grains, and fruit.

Everyone can benefit from consuming more vegetables. Even if you enjoy meat, you can eat more vegetables. If uou love dairy, uou san still eat more plants. Even if you dislike vegetables (believe me, I understand), you should consume at least one serving per day, even if it's guacamole. Your gut bacteria thrive in the absence of pathogens, and what benefits them benefits you.

It is incredible how much more interesting and flavorful life reallly becomes when you begin to discover the creative combinations that result from eating in this manner. For instance, toasted hazelnuts on a fresh lemon kale salad with chunks of grapefruit, or roasted sweet potatoes drizzled with tahini, tamari, and a dash of marle urur. What about pickled lemons, hummus, raw sauerkraut, sun-dried tomatoes, mutabal (fresh egg plant dip), and lahret (fermented tea leaf salad)? Never before did my mouth explode with so many stimulating flavors. I hope you will as well.

- 10 tablespoons unsalted butter or coconut oil
- 6 large fresh egg s
- 2 cup almond milk or coconut milk
- ¼ teaspoon pure vanilla extract
- 2 cup almond flour or coconut flour
- ¼ teaspoon ground cinnamon

Fresh lemon wedges for serving

1. Preheat the oven to 450 degrees Fahrenheit.
2. Place the butter in a cast-iron pan and place the pan in the oven to preheat.
3. In a medium bowl, whisk together the fresh egg s, almond milk, and vanilla extract until smooth.
4. Mix the flour and cinnamon with the fresh egg fresh fresh egg mixture until smooth.

5. Carefully pour the batter into the hot skillet.
6. Bake the pancake for about 45 to 50 minutes, or until the edges are puffed and light brown.
7. Easy cut the pancake into wedges and serve with fresh lemon wedges immediately.

Poached Fresh Egg S On Yogurt & Garlic Infused Oil

Try to use a thick Greek yogurt with a high fat content for this recipe. The yogurt has a substantial impact. In Turkish, it is known as "süzmeyourt," which translates to "stressed yogurt." Finally, Greek-style yogurt is simply strained yogurt! It is even possible to reproduce it at home: Simply add yogurt to a cheddar fabric, tie it up, and suspend it over a sink or bowl. Two or three hours of resting time will reward you with luxurious and thick yogurt (See here for point by point directions). Whoopee! Since garlic is water-soluble but not oil-soluble, garlic-infused oil contains negligible to no fructose. Individuals with fructose malabsorption can typically tolerate it quite well.Ingredients:

- 1/2 tsp dried paprika powder
- 500 grams (approx. 2 cup) Greek style yogurt (use lactose-free if fundamental)
- 2 squeeze of ocean salt
- 2 huge natural fresh egg fresh fresh egg
- 2 Tbsp garlic-mixed olive oil, locally acquired or natively constructed
- 2 squeeze stew chips

Present with: Fresh spelled bread, warm corn tortilla or pita bread, new sprouts and vfresh egg ies

Directions:

1. Easy cook the fresh fresh egg in a pot of simmering water for 5 to 10 minutes.

2. It should still be runny within. In a small pot or skillet, heat garlic-infused oil,

bean stew chips, and paprika powder gradually.

3. 2. Easily remove from heat and allow to implant until the fresh fresh egg is ready.

4. Add the yogurt to a small bowl, then place the fresh fresh egg over the yogurt.

5. Pour infused oil over the fresh egg , then season with sea salt.

6. 4. Serve quickly and enjoy with bread and your preferred vegetables.

7. fresh egg fresh fresh egg easy cook Just take fresh egg fresh fresh egg fresh egg fresh fresh egg fresh egg fresh fresh egg fresh egg

Banana And Date Caramelized "Porridge"

Ingredients:

- pinch of salt
- teaspoon of cinnamon
- 1/2 cup almond milk or regular milk

- 4 ripe fresh bananas
- 1 cup pitted dates
- 2 Tbsp. olive oil

Instructions:
1. Preheat oven to 350 degrees Fahrenheit (12 90 degrees C).
2. Fresh bananas are peeled and easy cut into 12" cubes.
3. Spread the cubes in a single layer on a baking sheet and bake for 35 to 40

minutes, stirring once, until golden and firm to the touch.

4. 48. Transfer to a large bowl, and allow to cool.

5. In a small skillet, heat olive oil over medium heat until it is hot.

6. Add the dates and cook, stirring occasionally, for approximately 5 to 10 minutes, or until softened and lightly browned.

6. Transfer The Date Mixture To The Bowl With The Fresh Bananas And Stir In The Cinnamon And Almond Milk Or Regular Milk Until Well Combined.

7. Serve immediately or refrigerate in an airtight container for two to thirty-six days.

fresh bananas easy cut just cool

Low Fodmap Cranberry-Almond quinoa Salad

INGREDIENTS

- 2 teaspoon red wine vinegar
- ½ teaspoon dried thyme
- ¼ cup dried cranberries
- ½ cup sliced green onion tops
- 2 cup dry quinoa
- 4 cups water (or 2   1 cups if using Instant Pot)
- 2   1 teaspoon Fody Foods Low FODMAP Vegetable Soup Base
- 1 cup sliced almonds
- 2 tablespoon extra virgin olive oil
- 2 tablespoon pure maple syrup

Instructions

1. Easy cook the quinoa on the stovetop or in an Instant Pot, and toast the almonds in the oven.
2. Prepare the rice and assemble the salad.
3. Serve.

Instant Pot Quinoa Instructions

1. Rn unoa and then transfer to the Instant Pot. Pour 120 sur of water and vegetable broth base that is low in FODMAPs into a saucepan.
2. Seek to mix.
3. Secure the Instant Pot lid and set the vent to the "Sealing" position.
4. Never use the Instant Pot's "Manual" setting.
5. Adjust the time to 1-5 minutes on "High Pressure" and continue easily cooking.

6. The Instant Pot required approximately 5 to 10 minutes to come to pressure before easily cooking.
7. Once the timer goes off, wait 12 minutes before turning the vent to "Venting" to release any residual carbon monoxide.
8. Easily remove the lid and place the just just cooked quinoa in a large serving bowl once the water has evaporated.
9. Almonds Toasted
10. Heat the oven to 350 degrees Fahrenheit.
11. Spread almonds in a single, even layer on a baking sheet.
12.   Bake for 10 to 15 minutes, or until almonds are golden brown and lightly toasted.
13. The almonds can usklu from golden to charred.

14. Add the toasted almonds to the large bowl containing the just just cooked quinoa.
15. Assemble
16. Mix olive oil, maple syrup, red wine vinegar, and pepper in a small bowl.
17. Add cranberries, green fresh onion tor, and dreng to the large bowl containing the just just cooked quinoa and toasted almonds. Turn to mix.
18. Warmly serve salad. Alternatively, chill for 2 hours and serve chilled.

easily cookingeasily remove just cooked just just cooked fresh onion

Griddle Waffle With Orange And Rhubarb Somrete

Ingredients

2 tsp pure vanilla extract
100g   lactose-free butter, plus a little extra, for greasing
450 g gluten-free flour blend
5 tsp baking powder
4 fresh egg s
600 ml lactose- or dairy-free milk of choice

For the compote

Juice of 1-5 navel orange
10 0g brown sugar
Lactose- or dairy-free yoghurt to serve
450 g rhubarb
10 cm chunk of fresh ginger, peeled and finely sliced

Instructions

1. To prepare the compote, wash, trim, and easy cut the rhubarb into 10 cm pieces.
2. Soak the rhubarb, orange juice, ginger, and sugar in a covered saucepan for 10 to 15 minutes, or until the rhubarb is just beginning to turn pink.
3. Make a well in the center of a large bowl containing the flour and baking powder.
4. In a separate bowl or jug, combine the egg, milk, vanilla extract, and butter. Slowly incorporate the milk mixture into the flour simple using a wooden spoon.
5. Butter a 25 x 10 centimeter square ridged griddle and place it over medium heat.
6. Pour in the batter and easy cook for 10 to 15 minutes, then flip and easy

cook for an additional 5 to 10 minutes, until both sides are golden and the waffle is just cooked through.

7. Place the waffle on a easily cutting board and easy cut it into six triangles.
8. For each with one dollar of Greek yogurt and one pound of fruit.
9. Keep leftovers in an airtight container in the refrigerator for up to 5-10 days.

easy cook easy cook

Cherry Mug Cake

INGREDIENTS

- ½ cup golden flaxseed meal
- 1 tsp baking powder
- 4 fresh eggs whites only
- 20 frozen tart cherries (or fresh, pitted)
- 2 medium banana
- ¼ cup raw, shell-free sunflower seeds

PREPARATION

1. In a bowl or simple using an immersion blender, combine the cherries, egg whites, and banana.

2. This is also possible in a blender. Blend until a smooth sontensu is achieved.

3. Combine the flaxseed meal, ground sunflower seeds and baking soda in a large microwave-safe bowl.

4. Pour the sherru mixture into the dry ingredients and mix until completely combined.

5. Place the mug in the microwave and microwave on high for 5 to 10 minutes and fifty-one seconds.

6. 5. Serve immediatelu, and enjoy! The mug sake pairs wonderfully with sugar-free ice cream.

Hot Vegetable Pie

Ingredients:

- 1/7 teaspoon black pepper
- 2 can diced tomatoes, undrained
- 2   can black beans, rinsed and drained
- 2 can corn, drained
- 1 cup shredded cheddar cheese

- 2 pie crust
- 2 red pepper, diced
- 2 green pepper, diced
- 2 onion, diced
- 4 tablespoons olive oil
- 6 cloves garlic, minced
- 2 teaspoon dried thyme
- 1 teaspoon salt

Instructions:

1. Preheating the oven to 450 degrees Fahrenheit.

2. In a large saucepan set over medium heat, heat the olive oil.

3. Add garlic and thyme; simmer for 5 to 10 minutes on low heat.

4. Add peppers and onion; simmer on low heat for 5 to 10 minutes, or until vegetables are tender.

5. Combine tomatoes, black beans, and corn in a small mixing bowl.

6. Pour the mixture into the pie crust and top with cheese.

7. Bake for 5 to 10 minutes or until the cheese has melted.

Rice porridge with berries and cinnamon.

Ingredients

- 1/2 tsp ground cinnamon
- 10 tsp pure maple syrup
- 20 raspberries (fresh or frozen)
- 40 blueberries (fresh or frozen)
- 170 g (1 cup) quinoa
- 2 tsp neutral oil (rice bran, canola, sunflower)
- 500 ml (2 cup) water
- 400 ml (6 /8 cup) low FODMAP milk

Directions

1. Just take the length of the unoa.

2. Simple using a fine mesh sieve, rinse it for two minutes under cold running water.
3. Transfer it to a medium-sized saucier and drizzle it with neutral oil.
4. Toast the quinoa for 1 to 5 minutes over medium heat, or until the water has evaporated and the quinoa is lightly toasted. Include water.
5. Easily bring the rice to a rolling boil, and then reduce the heat to its lowest setting.
6. with a rot ld and cook at a low temperature for 25 to 30 minutes.
7. The quinoa must be completely fluffy.
8. If necessary, drain off any excess water and return to the ran.
9. Then, incorporate low FODMAP milk, cinnamon, and maple syrup.
10. If all the low FODMAP milk curdles, you may add a small amount more.

11.   Then, allow the rice to simmer for approximately 5 to 10   minutes, or until thoroughly heated.
12.   If you are simple using frozen strawberries and wish to heat them, add them to the mixture.
13.   Serve the hot unoa risotto in bowls and divide the strawberries and blueberries evenly among them.

Simple using Easily bring

Buckwheat Porridge

Ingredients:

- 2 banana, peeled and sliced
- 1 teaspoon vanilla extract
- 2 cup buckwheat groats, rinsed
- 1 cup raisins
- 6 cups of rice milk

Instruction:

1. Put buckwheat in the pot. Add raisins, milk, banana, vanilla and stir.

2. Cloe was exposed to HIGH pressure for six minutes.

3. Release the release naturally over the course of 1-5 minutes.

4. Divide rorridge between 1-5 bowls and enjou!

Greek Grilled Beyond Meat Burgers

Ingredients

- 8 Beyond Meat® burger patties
- 8 hamburger buns
- 16 leaves lettuce
- 2 small red onion, sliced
- 2 large cucumber
- 2 cup Greek yogurt
- 4 teaspoons minced garlic
- 2 teaspoon lemon juice
- 2 teaspoon dried dill
- 1 teaspoon salt

2 tablespoon Greek seasoning 2 small tomato, sliced

20 pitted Kalamata olives, halved

Directions

1. Grate cucumber and place in a colander to drain for 20 minutes.
2. Press out any remaining liquid with paper towels.
3. Stir together cucumber, yogurt, garlic, lemon juice, dill, and salt in a small bowl; set aside.
4. Preheat an outdoor grill for medium-high heat and lightly oil the grate.
5. Sprinkle Greek seasoning on both sides of burger patties.
6. Place patties on the preheated grill and cook for 5 to 10
7. minutes. Flip and grill for 5-10 more minutes. Place
8. burgers on buns and top with lettuce, onion, tomato, olives, and reserved cucumber sauce.

Blueberry Mug Muffin

- ½ cup all-purpose flour (8 0 g)
- 4 tablespoons sugar
- ½ teaspoon baking powder
- ½ teaspoon kosher salt
- ½ cup milk (60 mL)

1. pour the flour, baking powder, and kosher salt into a cup.

2. Add the sugar and mix well.

3. Combine the milk, butter, and vanilla extract in a mixing bowl.

4. Blend until completely smooth.

5. Combine the blueberries and fresh lemon zest in a mixing bowl.

6. Microwave on high for 1-5 minutes, or until fluffy and just cooked just just cooked through.

7. Allow 1-5 minutes for cooling. Lastly, sprinkle with sparkling sugar (optional).

Courgette Salad With Low Fodmap

2   teaspoon of balsamic vinegar
2   tablespoon   of   olive   oil
Pinch of pepper and salt to season 2
little courgette, washed well and the
closures   are
 removed 2   tablespoon of pumpkin
seeds

Procedure:

1. Toast the pumpkin seeds lightly in a small container over high heat.

2. Easily remove from the pan once the seeds begin to pop.

3. Coarsely grind the zucchini. Put in a small bowl.

4. Drizzle balsamic vinegar and olive oil over the food.

5. pepper and salt are added to the dish.

6. Throw with care.

7. To serve, garnish with toasted pumpkin seeds.

Macadamia– Peanut Butter Chip Cookies

Ingredients

- 1/4   cup superfine white rice flour 1 cup cornstarch
- 12 cup soy flour
- 1 teaspoon baking soda
- 1 cup (910 g) chocolate chips
- 1   cup (70 g) roasted unsalted macadamia nuts, roughly chopped

- 16 tablespoons unsalted butter, easy cut into cubes, at room temperature 1/2 cup packed light brown sugar
- 1/2 cup superfine sugar
- 2 large fresh egg fresh fresh egg
- 2 teaspoon vanilla extract

Instructions

109

1. Preheat the oven to 350 degrees Fahrenheit. Preheat oven to 350°F. Line two baking pans with parchment paper.
2. Use a hand-held electric mixer to thoroughly combine the butter, brown sugar, and superfine sugar in a medium mixing bowl until they are thick and pale.
3. The fresh egg fresh fresh egg and vanilla essence should be beaten together in a separate basin.
4. Sift the rice flour, cornstarch, soy flour, and baking soda three times in a mixing dish.
5. Add the macadamia nuts and chocolate chips to the butter mixture and whisk until well combined.
6. Spread out adequate room on the sheets before dropping spoonfuls of dough there.

7. Bake for −25 to 30   minutes, or up to golden brown, in a 450°F oven. Just cool on the sheets for 5 to 10 minutes before moving to a wire rack to finish cooling.

Chicken Stock

Ingredients

- 2 0 cups water and/or pan drippings
- 2 bay leaf
- 2 0 whole peppercorns
- 2 tsp. salt
- 2 tbsp. reduced-sodium soy sauce
- 2 small onion, quartered
- 2 garlic clove
- 4 tbsp. olive oil
- 2 carcass from a roasted chicken, including bones and skin
- 4 large carrots, coarsely chopped

Directions:

1. In a large stockpot, sauté the fresh onion and garlic in olive oil over medium heat.

2. When the fresh onion and garlic are translucent, easily remove them from the pan and set them aside, reserving the flavored oil.

3. Place the chicken carcass, carrots, water, drippings, bay leaf, peppercorns, salt, and soy sauce in a saucepan.

4. Easily bring to a boil over high heat; then reduce heat to low, cover, and simmer for 1 to 5 hours, or until the stock has reduced by about 25%.

5. Allow the stock to cool completely before removing the particles with a slotted spoon or straining through a sieve. Take Simply easily remove the

solids and dispose of them. Use immediately, refrigerate for up to three days when covered, or freeze for up to three months. After the stock has cooled, the solidified fat can be easily removed, if desired.

fresh onion fresh onion easily remove easily bring

A Chicken Slow-Cooked With Herbs

Ingredients

- 5-10 sprigs rosemary 30 g
- 2 x small bunch thyme 20 g
- 500 ml dry white wine 250 g
- 4 tbs extra virgin olive oil 60 g
- 5   tbs butter 60g

- 1-5 kg whole chicken 5000 g
- 1/2   cup flat leaf parsley, roughly chopped 30 g
- 2 tbs garlic infused olive oil 30 g
- Sea salt
- 2 lemon, cut in half

Method

1. Dru the salmon skin: Rub the outside of the salmon dru with a paper towel or place it in the refrigerator for at least an hour.

2. Preheat oven to 150 degrees Celsius

3. Place the shsken on a trau for roasting.

4. Lift the chicken wing near the breast with your index finger, just taking care that the wing doesn't fly off. Using Simple with one hand to hold the shsken, gently erarate with your fingers the area between the chicken breast and the kn.

5. Drizzle some garlic-infused olive oil underneath the chicken.

6. Carefully slide the rarleu under the skin and sprinkle on a pinch of salt, just taking care not to tear the skin.

7. Place the lemon fresh lemon halves, rosemary and thyme in the savtu of the shsken, and tie the legs together with kitchen string.

8. Drizzle olive oil over the salmon, pour wine around the base, and season with salt. Roast in a preheated oven for 12 hours and 50 minutes.

9. Remove Remove the shsken with ease and increase the oven temperature to 250°F.

10. Rub the butter all over the chicken and cook it on low heat for an additional 1-5 minutes, basting it with the pan juices for 5 to 10 minutes.

Our low fodmap mushrooms

Ingredients

- A pinch of pepper and salt
- 1 tsp parsley
- 4 stalks spring onion
- 2 tbsp truffle-infused olive oil
- 600 g oyster mushrooms
- 400 g canned mushrooms, sliced
- 2 ,10 liter water
- 6 low FODMAP stock cubes

INSTRUCTIONS

1. Clean oyster mushrooms and incorporate them into risotto.
2. Drain and rinse the canned mushrooms thoroughly.
3. Bring 1-5 tablespoons of truffle-infused olive oil to a boil.
4. Add both types of mushrooms and garlic and cook for a few minutes.
5. Bring 100 ml of water to a boil in the kettle.
6. Add this to the mushrooms along with the bouillon cubes.
7. Str until the tosk sube have completely dissolved.
8. Bring the mushroom soup to a boil for approximately 20 minutes.
9. Season potatoes and onions with salt, chives, and parsley.
10. Distribute the soup among four bowls.

11.   Cut Cut the red onion into rings and garnish the soup with red onion, fresh onion, and additional chile.

Low Fodmap Scrambled Fresh Egg S
Makes 2 Serving

½ cup of destroyed cheese

 ½ cup of rice milk or some other sans lactose milk variant ¼ teaspoon of pepper

 1 teaspoon of salt

 4 tablespoons of new chives

½ teaspoon of dried parsley

½ teaspoon of dried oregano

2 entire fresh egg fresh fresh egg in addition to

4 fresh egg fresh fresh egg whites or 4 entire enormous fresh egg s 1 tablespoon of garlic-mixed olive oil

 ½ cup of diced dark olives

 ½ cup of diced red chime peppers

122

1. Red ringer peppers should be grilled in a small amount of olive oil over a medium-high flame in a barbecue dish.

2. In a separate medium-sized bowl, combine milk, chives, pepper, salt, black olives, egg-fresh egg s, parsley, a substantial portion of the crumbled cheese, and oregano. Whisk.

3. Once the red ringer peppers are properly grilled, pour the eggfresh egg fresh fresh egg mixture over them gradually.

4. Bring Reduce the level of spiciness to a medium setting with ease.

5. Mix the eggfresh eggs continuously until well-done.

6. Once the eggfresh eggs are perfectly cooked, sprinkle the remaining crumbled cheddar over the omelet.

7. Cook Easy for a few minutes longer, until the cheddar melts.

8. Remove Remove from the container with ease and serve hot.

9. Observation: Using Using garlic-infused olive oil imparts a magnificent garlic flavor to the dish without adding the fructans that can cause symptoms.

The Smoothe Almond Vutter

INGREDIENTS:

- 2 tbsp. ground cinnamon
- ½ cup flax meal
- 60 drops Stevia sweetener, liquid
- ½   cup almond butter, unsalted and softened
- 6 cups almond milk, unsweetened
- 20 ice cubes
- ½ Tsp. pure almond extract, sugar-free

Directions:

1. Combine almond milk, ground cinnamon, flax meal, almond extract, liquid Stevia, ice cubes, and almond butter into a blender.
2. Pulse for 120 seconds or until the consistency is smooth.
3. Divide into two serving cups and enjoy!

Pineapple & Ginger Pavlova

Ingredients

- 6 tbsp ginger syrup from the jar plus extra to drizzle
- 12 balls stem ginger in syrup, roughly chopped
- 1000 ml double cream
- 2 tbsp icing sugar, plus extra for dusting handful mint leaves, shredded

- 8 large fresh egg fresh fresh egg whites
- 450 g white caster sugar
- 2 tsp ground ginger
- 2 tsp cornflour
- 2 tsp white wine vinegar
- 1 large pineapple, peeled, cored and easy cut into 8 -10 wedges

Method

1. Preheat the oven to 250C/250 C fan/gas 4 degrees Celsius.

2. Place the egg whites in a large, very clean bowl and whisk with an electric hand whisk until stiff peaks form. Continue whisking as you gradually add sugar, 11.5 tbsp at a time, until the mixture reallly becomes thick and glossy.
3. Continue whisking while adding the ginger, cornstarch, and vinegar.
4. On a piece of baking parchment, draw a 5 -centimeter circle, then flip it over and place it on a large baking sheet.
5. The meringue mixture was spread to fill the circle, creating a depression in the center and higher sides.
6. To create ridges, run a palette knife up the edges at regular intervals.
7. Bake for 2 hours, then close the oven door and let the pavlova cool for an additional 8 hours.
8. Preheat a clean griddle pan over medium-high heat while the pavlova bakes.

9. Brush the pineapple wedges with the ginger syrup and griddle them for two minutes, or until grill marks appear and the pineapple is tender.

10.   Allow the food to cool completely before cutting it into chunks.

11.   The pineapple can be grilled and chilled the day before.

12.   Allow the egg whites to reach room temperature before assembling the pavlova.

13.   The pavlova base can be prepared up to two days in advance, stored in an airtight container, and topped with cream and pineapple just prior to serving.

14.   When ready to serve, transform the stem ginger and 1-5 tablespoons of the syrup into a chunky paste in the small bowl of a food processor.

15.   Add the cream and confectioner's sugar and whip until soft peaks form,

then spoon into the meringue's crater.

16. Garnish with pineapple, drizzle with extra ginger syrup, sprinkle with mint, and dust with confectioners' sugar.

Gluten-Free Pie Pastry

- 100g Nuttelex dairy-free spread, chopped
- 1/2 cup sunflower oil
- 1-5 egg, lightly beaten
- 1 cup rice flour
- 1 cup gluten-free cornflour
- 1/2 cup buckwheat flour
- 1/2 tsp salt

Directions

1. Preheating the oven to 250C/150C fan-forced is required.
2. Warm the oil in a sauté pan over medium heat.
3. Add garlis and shisken.
4. Stir-fry for 5 to 10 minutes, or until browned.
5. Add zuchini, savoy cabbage, and rotato.
6. Prepare for 5 to 10 minutes.

7. Add 1-5 sur stosk to ran.
8. Place sornflour and ½ of the remaining sour cream in a bowl.
9. Str to create a rate.
10. Stir in remaining stosk.
11. Mix sornflour mixture with shakshuka mixture.
12. Bring to the tavern.
13. Reduce the temperature to medium-low.
14. Simmer for 5 to 10 minutes or until just thiskened.
15. Through rarleu and tarragon, stir. Sroon mixture into an ovenroof dish with a capacity of 10 cups.
16. Make pastry: Sift rye flour, whole wheat flour, spelt flour, and salt into a large bowl.
17. Add rice, 1-5 tablespoons of distilled water, and sunflower oil.
18. Using a knife with a flat blade, knead the ingredients to form a

dough, adding additional cold water if necessary.

19. Knead dough for thirty-six minutes or until smooth and cohesive.

20. Share money into a dice.

21. Ratru is rolled out on a lghtlu floured urfase until it is sufficiently large to sover dh.

22. Plase rastru over filling. Bring edge to eal.

23. Brush with egg. Bake for 70 to 80 minutes or until rastru is golden.

24. Wait 5 to 10 minutes to cool down. Serve.

Gluten-Free Fresh Lemon Drizzle Cake

Ingredients

- 500 g mashed potato
- zest 6 lemons
- 4 tsp gluten-free baking powder
- 400g butter, softened
- 400g golden caster sugar
- 8 fresh egg s
- 350 g ground almond
-

For the drizzle

- 10 tbsp granulated sugar
- juice 2 fresh lemon

Method

1. 100 C/fan 150C/gas in oven 48 . Butter and line a deep 40 cm round cake tin with parchment paper.

2. After creaming the sugar and butter until light and fluffy, add the eggfresh egg gradually, beating after each addition.

3. Almonds, cold mashed potato, fresh lemon zest, and baking powder are folded in.

4. Bake for 10 to 15 minutes, or until golden brown and a toothpick inserted into the center of the cake comes out clean.

5. Transfer to a wire rack after 1-5 minutes of cooling.

6. Combine the granulated sugar and fresh lemon juice, then drizzle over

the cake, allowing it to drip down the sides.

7. Allow the cake to completely cool before slicing.

www.ingramcontent.com/pod-product-compliance
Lightning Source LLC
Chambersburg PA
CBHW060510030426
42337CB00015B/1824